NON-SURGICAL FACELIFT METHODS FOR BEGINNERS

Effective Techniques For Wrinkle Reduction, Skin Tightening, And Youthful Radiance Without Surgery

DR SAWYER DIEGO

TABLE OF CONTENTS

ABOUT THE BOOK

"Non-Surgical Facelift Methods for Beginners" is an invaluable resource for anyone looking for safe and efficient substitutes for conventional surgical facelift procedures. Everyone wants to age gracefully, and this book tackles the rising trend of non-surgical facelift techniques by offering thorough explanations of their advantages and real-world applications.

This book explores the nuances of aging, from the gradual loss of skin elasticity to the development of fine lines and wrinkles, emphasizing the critical role that facial muscle tone and skin health play in maintaining a youthful appearance. Facial aging is a natural process that is influenced by various factors, including genetics, lifestyle choices, and environmental exposures.

This book carefully sorts and explains the wide variety of non-surgical facelift techniques that are currently on the market, such as threads, lasers, and radiofrequency treatments.

It breaks down each technique to show how it works differently to address particular facial issues like loss of volume, uneven texture, and sagging skin. It also looks closely at the advantages and possible drawbacks of each technique so that readers can make well-informed decisions based on their requirements and expectations.

Choosing a procedure alone is not enough to prepare for a non-surgical facelift; careful planning and consideration are needed. This book walks readers through every stage of the pre-procedure phase, from initial consultations with specialists to financial planning and mental preparation. It also offers helpful advice on skin care routines, post-procedure care, and long-term maintenance, ensuring that readers can maximize recovery and longevity of results.

A comprehensive understanding of what it entails to undergo non-surgical facelift procedures is provided by exploring the legal considerations, patient rights, and financial implications.

Potential risks and complications associated with these procedures are also addressed in detail, emphasizing the importance of minimizing risks through proper technique and vigilant aftercare.

This book explores emerging trends in non-invasive facial rejuvenation, potential breakthroughs in skincare, and the fusion of holistic approaches with modern methodologies. As the field of non-surgical facelifts continues to evolve, it looks ahead to future trends and advancements in technology and technique. By staying informed about these advancements, readers are encouraged to remain proactive in their journey toward achieving and maintaining youthful facial aesthetics.

CHAPTER ONE

NON-SURGICAL FACELIFT METHODS OVERVIEW

WHAT ARE TECHNIQUES FOR NON-SURGICAL FACELIFTS?

The term "non-surgical facelift methods" refers to a range of minimally invasive cosmetic procedures that are intended to rejuvenate the face without the need for invasive surgery. These procedures include dermal fillers, such as hyaluronic acid injections, which are used to restore volume to areas that have lost firmness and elasticity due to aging; Botox injections, which target wrinkles by relaxing muscles that cause lines and creases, especially around the forehead and eyes; laser treatments, such as intense pulsed light (IPL) or laser resurfacing, help improve skin texture, tone, and pigmentation issues; and thread lifts, which entail inserting dissolvable threads under the skin to lift and tighten sagging facial tissues.

Understanding these techniques is essential for anyone considering facial rejuvenation, as they offer effective alternatives to surgery with fewer complications and quicker recovery times. Each method targets specific aging concerns and provides noticeable results with minimal downtime compared to surgical facelifts.

Non-surgical techniques are popular because they can enhance facial appearance without the risks and recovery period associated with surgery. They offer a customizable approach, allowing individuals to target precise areas of concern and achieve natural-looking results.

ADVANTAGES OF SURGICAL CHOICES

Compared to traditional surgical facelifts, non-surgical facelift methods have several advantages. Firstly, they require little to no recovery time, so patients can get back to their regular activities right away. This is especially convenient for people who lead busy lives and cannot afford to take time off for recovery. Secondly, non-surgical facelifts are less invasive, which lowers the risk of complications like scarring or infection. Finally, non-surgical facelifts are typically less expensive than surgical options, making facial rejuvenation accessible to a wider range of people.

The ability to achieve gradual improvements is another important advantage of non-surgical methods. As the skin responds to treatments such as fillers or collagen-stimulating procedures, results usually show up gradually over several weeks.

This natural progression allows for adjustments to be made to achieve the desired outcome without the immediate, dramatic change that is often associated with surgery. Additionally, non-surgical facelift methods can be combined with other cosmetic procedures to further enhance results, offering a comprehensive approach to facial rejuvenation tailored to individual needs and preferences.

WHO QUALIFIES FOR NON-SURGICAL FACELIFT BENEFITS?

Non-surgical facelift techniques are appropriate for people who wish to enhance non-surgically the appearance of fine lines, wrinkles, sagging skin, and loss of facial volume.

Those who are in good general health and have reasonable expectations about the results of non-surgical procedures are the best candidates. These techniques are especially helpful for younger patients who want to avoid or postpone the need for surgery, as well as older people who want to rejuvenate their appearance without the risks and recovery associated with surgery.

In addition, non-surgical facelift techniques are a great option for people who would rather take their time rejuvenating their faces or who are worried about the possible negative effects of surgery.

They also allow for customized treatment plans that address individual aesthetic goals and offer flexibility in targeting specific areas of concern. It is important to consult with a qualified cosmetic practitioner to determine whether a patient is a good candidate for non-surgical facelift techniques based on their skin condition, medical history, and desired outcomes.

THE VALUE OF SAFE PRACTICE AND CORRECT METHODOLOGY

The significance of appropriate technique and safety in non-surgical facelift methods cannot be emphasized. While non-surgical procedures do not require precise surgical skills, they still require expertise and a comprehensive understanding of facial anatomy.

Practitioners who wish to ensure safe and effective outcomes for their patients must be trained and certified in the administration of treatments like thread lifts, lasers, and injectables.

Safe protocols, including sterile techniques and appropriate equipment, are crucial to minimize the risk of infection and ensure patient comfort throughout the procedure. This lowers the risk of complications such as bruising, allergic reactions, or asymmetry by ensuring that treatments are delivered precisely to target areas without causing damage to surrounding tissues or nerves.

In addition, patients and practitioners must be aware of the drawbacks and possible adverse effects of each non-surgical technique.

Practitioners should also inform patients about what to anticipate both during and after treatment, including possible temporary swelling, bruises, or mild discomfort.

Stressing safety and appropriate techniques not only improves treatment outcomes but also fosters patient-provider trust, which guarantees a positive experience and satisfactory outcomes.

AN OVERVIEW OF THE EXPECTATIONS FOR THIS BOOK

Readers will obtain a thorough understanding of various non-invasive techniques, including dermal fillers, Botox injections, laser treatments, and thread lifts, along with their benefits and potential risks. Detailed explanations and step-by-step instructions will help readers navigate the process of choosing the right treatments based on their individual aesthetic goals and concerns.

This book offers a comprehensive guide to non-surgical facelift methods, offering practical insights and expert advice for beginners interested in facial rejuvenation.

Apart from the procedural details, this book encompasses crucial subjects like eligibility requirements, pre-treatment preparation, recuperation techniques, and long-term maintenance plans. Readers will discover the significance of choosing certified professionals, safety factors, and reasonable expectations for outcomes. By providing readers with useful information and understanding, this book seeks to enable people to make knowledgeable decisions regarding non-surgical facelift procedures and attain safe and efficient natural-looking facial rejuvenation.

CHAPTER TWO

FUNDAMENTALS OF FACIAL CHANGES AND AGING

RECOGNIZING THE IMPACT OF AGING ON FACE APPEARANCE

Our facial appearance changes noticeably as we age due to a variety of physiological processes. One of the main causes of facial aging is the progressive loss of collagen and elastin, which are proteins that give skin its elasticity and firmness.

This loss results in wrinkles, fine lines, and sagging skin, especially around the mouth, forehead, and eyes. As we age, the volume of our facial bones and fat pads also decreases, changing the contours of our face and making it appear more hollowed out.

Sun exposure also contributes significantly to aging because UV radiation damages the skin's structure over time, resulting in the formation of age spots, uneven skin tone, and the breakdown of collagen fibers.

In addition, lifestyle factors like smoking and poor nutrition can hasten the aging process by increasing inflammation and oxidative stress in the body, which in turn affects the health of the skin overall.

For those who are interested in using non-surgical facelift methods to address signs of aging, it is important to understand these processes. By understanding how aging affects facial appearance, people can better appreciate the underlying mechanisms that non-surgical treatments seek to counteract. These insights enable people to make well-informed decisions about their skincare regimens and available treatments, ensuring they get the best results possible that are customized to their individual needs and concerns.

TYPICAL AGING SYMPTOMS AND THEIR CAUSES

Several common signs of aging that are visible on the face are internal changes that are happening within the skin and underlying structures; the first to show signs of aging are fine lines and wrinkles, which deepen with time due to repeated facial movements and a reduction in collagen production. These lines are especially noticeable in areas of the face that are frequently expressed, like the forehead and the area around the eyes (crow's feet).

In addition to causing sagging skin and the development of jowls, loss of facial volume and elasticity also weakens collagen and elastin fibers and reduces facial fat pads, which changes the shape of the jawline and cheeks.

Age spots also referred to as liver spots or sunspots, are caused by prolonged sun exposure and result in localized pigmentation changes on the skin.

These signs of aging have many different causes, both extrinsic and intrinsic. Extrinsic factors include pollution, UV radiation, and lifestyle choices that cause oxidative stress and inflammation in the skin, which accelerates aging. Intrinsic aging is a natural process determined by genetics and hormonal changes that affect the skin's ability to regenerate and maintain its youthful appearance.

For those who are thinking about non-surgical facelift procedures, it is important to comprehend these typical symptoms and their underlying causes. By recognizing particular issues such as wrinkles, sagging skin, and age spots, patients can customize their treatment regimens to effectively address these problems. This information enables patients to select non-invasive procedures that are appropriate and rejuvenate their appearance.

RELEVANCE OF SKIN ELASTICITY AND FACIAL MUSCLE TONE

Skin elasticity and facial muscle tone are essential for looking young and avoiding obvious signs of aging. The firmness and resilience of facial muscles support the skin above it and help shape the face; as we age, these muscles weaken and lose tone, which causes drooping and sagging in areas like the jawline and cheeks.

Conversely, skin elasticity is the capacity of the skin to stretch and retract. Elasticity is mainly preserved by the collagen and elastin fibers in the dermis, which offer flexibility and structural support. As we age, our skin loses its production of these proteins, making it more prone to wrinkles and folds.

To achieve a natural-looking result with non-surgical facelift methods, it is important to maintain optimal facial muscle tone and skin elasticity.

Certain muscle groups can be targeted by facial exercises, which can help strengthen underlying muscles and improve overall facial contour. Moreover, collagen production-stimulating treatments like ultrasound and radiofrequency therapies enhance skin elasticity and firmness, promoting a more youthful appearance.

By focusing on enhancing muscle tone and restoring skin elasticity, individuals can achieve long-lasting results that rejuvenate their appearance and boost their confidence.

People can choose non-surgical facelift methods that effectively address their specific concerns by understanding the interplay between facial muscle tone and skin elasticity.

FACTORS AFFECTING THE AGING FACE

Genetic predispositions and hormonal fluctuations are examples of intrinsic factors that are unique to each individual and have an impact on facial aging. Genetic factors also determine the rate at which collagen and elastin fibers degrade, which affects skin thickness and resilience.

Hormonal fluctuations, especially during menopause, can accelerate the aging process by reducing collagen production and changing skin hydration levels.

Extrinsic factors—such as lifestyle choices and environmental exposures—also contribute significantly to the aging of the face. One of the main extrinsic factors is prolonged sun exposure, which causes photoaging—a condition marked by wrinkles, uneven pigmentation, and loss of skin elasticity. UV radiation accelerates the aging processes of the skin by damaging collagen fibers and promoting the formation of free radicals.

In addition to environmental factors like pollution and severe weather, lifestyle choices like smoking, eating poorly, and using insufficient skincare products aggravate the effects of oxidative stress on the skin by impairing its ability to regenerate and repair itself.

To effectively target specific concerns with non-invasive techniques that support long-term skin rejuvenation and maintenance, people seeking to mitigate the effects of facial aging through non-surgical facelift methods must understand the variety of factors influencing this process. By addressing both intrinsic and extrinsic factors, people can develop comprehensive skincare routines and treatment plans that promote skin health and vitality.

WHY POPULAR NON-SURGICAL FACELIFT TECHNIQUES

Techniques like dermal fillers, which restore lost volume and smooth wrinkles, offer immediate improvements in facial contour and skin texture. Non-surgical facelift methods have become more and more popular because they are effective at rejuvenating facial appearance without the risks and downtime associated with invasive surgical procedures. These methods appeal to people seeking natural-looking results with minimal discomfort and shorter recovery times.

The fact that non-surgical facelift techniques can treat multiple signs of aging at once is another factor in their popularity. For example, microcurrent therapy and laser skin resurfacing improve skin tone and stimulate collagen production, treating issues like sagging skin, fine lines, and uneven pigmentation all in one session. This all-encompassing approach enables patients to achieve harmonious facial rejuvenation customized to their own aesthetic goals.

Furthermore, non-surgical facelift techniques are frequently less expensive than conventional surgical methods, which open them up to a wider spectrum of people seeking cosmetic improvements. The fact that these procedures can be completed in the comfort of one's own home during office visits, without requiring general anesthesia or extended hospital stays, adds to their allure for active individuals and busy professionals.

In general, non-surgical facelift techniques are becoming more and more popular due to advances in cosmetic technology and consumer demand for safe and effective anti-aging solutions. People who opt for non-invasive techniques can attain results that are natural-looking, enhancing their facial features and restoring youthful vitality, thereby boosting their confidence and overall well-being.

CHAPTER THREE

DIFFERENT NON-SURGICAL FACELIFT TECHNIQUES

SUMMARY OF THE VARIOUS NON-SURGICAL ALTERNATIVES AVAILABLE

Non-surgical facelift techniques provide a variety of options for improving facial contours, tightening skin, and minimizing wrinkles without requiring invasive surgery. Dermal fillers, which use injectable substances like hyaluronic acid to plump areas of the face and smooth out wrinkles, are among the most popular techniques. Microcurrent therapy is another popular technique that uses low-level electrical currents to stimulate facial muscles, toning and lifting the skin.

Moreover, non-ablative laser treatments employ laser energy to enhance skin texture and promote collagen production, which is appropriate for decreasing age spots and fine lines. Radiofrequency treatments, on the other hand, apply heat energy to the skin's deeper layers, encouraging collagen tightening and remodeling. These procedures are attractive because they have less recovery time than surgery and little downtime, making them accessible options for people looking for non-invasive facial rejuvenation.

COMPARING DIFFERENT TECHNIQUES: RADIOFREQUENCY, THREADS, LASERS,

When thinking about non-surgical facelift techniques, it's important to know how each method functions and what results you hope to achieve.

Thread lifting is one technique that works well for mild to moderate facial sagging because it uses dissolvable threads inserted under the skin to lift sagging areas and gradually stimulate collagen production.

Conversely, laser treatments use a variety of light wavelengths to address particular skin concerns, such as uneven pigmentation, fine lines, and texture problems. Skin resurfacing and collagen stimulation can be achieved with lasers such as fractional CO_2 or

Erbium YAG, which produce smoother, firmer skin throughout multiple treatment sessions.

Effective for improving skin laxity and enhancing facial contours without surgery, radiofrequency treatments (e.g., Thermage, Ultherapy) deliver heat deep into the skin to tighten existing collagen fibers and stimulate new collagen production. The intensity and recovery time of each technique varies, so careful consideration should be given to individual skin types, desired results, and recovery tolerance.

HOW PARTICULAR FACIAL CONCERNS ARE TARGETED BY EACH METHOD

Based on their mechanisms of action, non-surgical facelift techniques are customized to address different types of facial concerns. For example, dermal fillers work best to restore youthful contours and add volume to areas like the lips, cheeks, and area around the mouth; microcurrent therapy targets the muscles in the face, improving tone and firmness by increasing circulation and stimulating muscle activity, which gives the appearance of being lifted.

Radiofrequency treatments penetrate deeper layers of the skin to tighten lax tissue and redefine facial contours; these procedures are especially effective for mild to moderate skin laxity and aging signs. Laser treatments address pigmentation issues, fine lines, and uneven texture by promoting collagen production and encouraging skin renewal. Thread lifting specifically targets sagging skin by inserting absorbable threads beneath the skin's surface, lifting and supporting tissue over time.

ADVANTAGES AND POSSIBLE DRAWBACKS OF EVERY TECHNIQUE

Dermal fillers offer instant results with little downtime and temporary improvements in facial volume and contour; however, side effects may include temporary redness, swelling, or bruising at the injection site.

Each non-surgical facelift technique has unique advantages and possible drawbacks to take into account.

Laser treatments offer precise targeting of specific skin concerns with minimal discomfort; however, side effects such as temporary redness, swelling, or changes in skin pigmentation can occur after treatment. Microcurrent therapy is non-invasive and painless, promoting natural collagen production and muscle toning without downtime. Few people experience mild tingling or muscle sensitivity during treatment.

Though there is minimal downtime, thread lifting offers immediate lifting effects with minimal discomfort; side effects, such as bruising, swelling, or transient sensations of tightness, are possible, but they resolve within a few days of treatment. Radiofrequency treatments are effective for skin tightening and contouring, with gradual improvements visible over several months.

SELECTING THE APPROPRIATE APPROACH DEPENDING ON PERSONAL NEEDS

The best non-surgical facelift technique depends on the patient's skin concerns, desired results, and lifestyle. Dermal fillers are best for regaining lost volume and improving facial contours, microcurrent therapy is a non-invasive method for tightening the skin and toning the muscles, and laser treatments are best for treating specific skin problems like pigmentation and fine lines.

Though thread lifting offers immediate lifting effects and long-term collagen stimulation, it is best suited for individuals with mild to moderate facial sagging. Consulting with a qualified aesthetic practitioner is crucial to assess candidacy, discuss expected outcomes, and customize a treatment plan that suits individual needs and preferences. Radiofrequency treatments are effective for overall skin tightening and rejuvenation, making them suitable for individuals seeking gradual improvements in facial contours and skin laxity.

CHAPTER FOUR

GETTING READY FOR AN ALL-NATURAL FACELIFT

FIRST CONSULTATION WITH AN EXPERT

One of the most important things you can do to get ready for a non-surgical facelift is to schedule an initial consultation with a specialist. This consultation will take place at your convenience and will involve talking through your aesthetic goals and concerns with a qualified practitioner, usually a dermatologist or cosmetic surgeon who specializes in non-invasive procedures.

The specialist will evaluate your skin condition, facial anatomy, and general health to see if you are a good candidate for non-surgical facelift methods. They will also go over the various non-surgical options that are available, like dermal fillers, thread lifts, or laser treatments, and will help you understand the advantages and possible risks of each procedure.

Furthermore, the initial consultation offers you the chance to ask questions and get any doubts you may have answered. The specialist will realistically explain the expected results, taking into account your particular facial structure and skin type. They will also go over the procedure's duration, recovery process, and potential side effects. To ensure your safety and the efficacy of the treatment plan, you must be honest and upfront during this consultation. By the end of it, you should have a clear idea of what to expect both during and after the procedure, enabling you to make an informed decision about pursuing a non-surgical facelift.

PRE-PROCEDURE HEALTH AND SKIN CARE ISSUES

Preparing your skin and general health before a non-surgical facelift is essential for the best outcomes and reducing risks. Your specialist will provide detailed instructions based on your skin type and the procedure you select. Generally, this entails implementing a skincare routine that improves skin health and gets ready for treatment; this can involve using mild cleansers, moisturizers, and sunscreens to minimize sensitivity and improve skin texture; it can also involve avoiding excessive sun exposure and smoking, which can greatly improve skin health and overall healing after the procedure.

Health considerations are just as important; your specialist will go over your medical history and current medications to find any factors that might compromise the safety or results of the procedure; they may suggest lifestyle changes to support skin recovery, like eating a balanced diet and staying hydrated; if needed, they may also recommend supplements or medications to improve skin condition and speed up healing.

RECOGNIZING REASONABLE GOALS AND RESULTS

Understanding realistic expectations and outcomes is crucial when planning a non-surgical facelift.

Although non-surgical procedures can produce noticeable improvements in facial appearance, they are not without limitations. The specialist will discuss what is realistically achievable based on your unique anatomy and skin condition during your consultation. The elasticity of the skin, the severity of wrinkles or sagging, and the overall structure of your face will all play a role in the final results.

Managing expectations is key to satisfaction post-procedure; while non-surgical facelift methods can provide a rejuvenated appearance, they may not completely halt the natural aging process. By understanding these realistic outcomes, you can make an informed decision about whether a non-surgical facelift aligns with your aesthetic goals and expectations. Your specialist will explain the potential results of the chosen procedure, including how long the effects are expected to last and any maintenance treatments that may be necessary.

A LOOK INTO INSURANCE AND FINANCIAL PLANNING

The cost of non-surgical facelifts varies greatly based on the technique utilized, the experience of the specialist, and your location. The specialist will provide you with a detailed cost estimate during your initial consultation that includes the procedure fee, any facility charges, and any post-procedure medications or skincare products. They may also go over financing options or payment plans that can help you afford the treatment.

Financial planning guarantees that you can comfortably afford the procedure and any associated costs, allowing you to focus on achieving your desired results with peace of mind. Some non-surgical facelift methods may require multiple sessions or maintenance treatments, which can impact long-term costs. Additionally, check with your insurance provider to understand coverage policies; typically, cosmetic procedures are not covered unless deemed medically necessary.

GETTING READY MENTALLY AND HANDLING ISSUES

To mentally prepare for a non-surgical facelift, you should address any fears or anxieties you may have about the procedure. It's normal to feel nervous about cosmetic procedures, even non-invasive ones. The specialist will spend time during your consultation to talk through your concerns and answer any questions, reassuring you and giving you information to ease your mind. They will also go over the steps of the procedure in detail, from preparation to recovery, making you feel more prepared and confident.

Mental preparation also entails understanding the benefits the procedure can have on your confidence and self-esteem, visualizing the possible results, and discussing your reasons for seeking a non-surgical facelift with the specialist. Reaffirming your decision and bringing your expectations in line with reality can be achieved by practicing relaxation techniques like mindfulness or deep breathing.

CHAPTER FIVE

PROCEDURE DAY: WHAT TO ANTICIPATE

STEP-BY-STEP DISSECTION OF A NORMAL PROCESS

To ensure your comfort during a non-surgical facelift, your healthcare provider will first assess your skin condition and discuss your goals with you. After that, the treatment area is cleaned thoroughly, and depending on the method chosen, a topical numbing cream may be applied to ensure your comfort. The actual treatment involves applying specialized devices or injectables; for instance, radiofrequency or ultrasound therapy aims to stimulate collagen production deep within the skin, providing a lifting effect over time, while dermal fillers or neurotoxins are strategically administered to lift and smooth targeted areas, like the forehead or cheeks.

Follow post-procedure instructions carefully to maximize results and minimize discomfort or side effects. During the procedure, your provider will explain each step and make sure you are comfortable. After the procedure, they may apply soothing agents to the treated area to minimize any temporary redness or swelling.

CHOICES FOR ANESTHESIA AND PAIN RELIEF METHODS

A local anesthetic or topical numbing cream is usually all that is needed for non-surgical facelift procedures, so you won't need general anesthesia to be comfortable during the procedure. Topical numbing creams are applied before the procedure to minimize any sensations during treatment. Certain procedures, such as injectable treatments, may contain lidocaine in the product itself to further reduce discomfort during and immediately after the injections.

If pain management is a concern for you, talking through your options with your provider beforehand will help you decide which the best course of action is. Most patients find these procedures to be fairly tolerable, and any discomfort they may experience will usually be mild and transient. Your healthcare provider will put your comfort first and can make necessary adjustments to techniques to guarantee a positive experience.

TIME SPENT DURING THE PROCEDURE AND RECUPERATION

Non-surgical facelift procedures can take anywhere from 30 minutes to an hour, with injectable procedures taking less time and treatments like ultrasound therapy needing longer sessions to achieve the best results. The exact method chosen and the number of areas treated determine how long the procedure takes.

While there may be some redness or swelling after many non-surgical facelift procedures, recovery times vary but are generally shorter than those following surgical alternatives. Results often appear gradually over the next few days to weeks as collagen production increases or injectables settle into place.

INSTRUCTIONS FOR IMMEDIATE POST-PROCEDURE CARE

Using gentle skincare products to nurture your skin as it heals and adhering to specific care instructions after a non-surgical facelift procedure can help maximize results and minimize potential side effects. Your provider may recommend avoiding excessive heat or sun exposure for a few days. Applying cold compresses can help reduce swelling, and sleeping with your head elevated can help minimize any fluid retention.

To ensure optimal healing and results, your healthcare provider will provide detailed post-procedure care guidelines tailored to your specific treatment and skin type. In addition, you may be instructed to refrain from vigorous exercise or activities that could increase blood flow to the face immediately following treatment.

POSSIBLE IMMEDIATE IMPACTS AND STRATEGIES FOR HANDLING THEM

Depending on the procedure, mild redness, swelling, or bruising at the treatment site is normal after a non-surgical facelift.

These effects are usually transient and go away in a few days to a week. During the first 24 hours, applying cold compresses intermittently can help reduce swelling and discomfort.

Your provider may also suggest gentle massage or specific skincare products to help minimize bruising and promote healing.

By adhering to recommended aftercare practices, you can promote a smooth recovery and enjoy the rejuvenating benefits of your non-surgical facelift procedure. It's important to avoid touching or rubbing the treated area excessively and to follow your provider's guidelines for skincare and makeup application post-procedure.

If you experience any unexpected or prolonged side effects, like severe swelling or pain, contact your healthcare provider right away to ensure prompt evaluation and appropriate management.

CHAPTER SIX

RECUPERATION AND CARE AFTER PROCEDURE

LONG-TERM MAINTENANCE AND CARE OF THE OUTCOMES

Following a non-surgical facelift, maintaining a youthful appearance and skin health requires long-term care and maintenance of results. To keep your procedure's benefits going, you must follow certain guidelines and follow a consistent skincare routine. These include protecting your skin from sun exposure by using broad-spectrum sunscreen every day, abstaining from smoking and excessive alcohol use, and eating a nutritious, vitamin- and antioxidant-rich diet.

Apart from external maintenance, internal hydration is crucial for preserving skin elasticity and general health. Drinking lots of water aids in the removal of toxins from the body and hydrates the skin from the inside out.

Additionally, adding light facial massages and using skincare products that have been prescribed by your dermatologist or aesthetician can prolong and improve the outcomes of your non-surgical facelift. Finally, consistency is essential for obtaining and preserving the desired youthful appearance over an extended period.

HANDLING BRUISING, SWELLING, AND DISCOMFITURE

After a non-surgical facelift, it's important to control swelling, bruising, and discomfort for a seamless recovery. Mild to moderate swelling and bruising are common after the procedure, and these can be controlled with prescribed medications and cold compresses. You can also reduce swelling by elevating your head while you rest. To minimize discomfort and encourage healing, carefully follow your healthcare provider's post-procedure care instructions.

Your healthcare provider may prescribe over-the-counter pain relievers to ease discomfort.

You should refrain from physically demanding activities and facial massages in the first post-operative period to avoid aggravating swelling or bruises. As your body heals, you can reduce swelling and bruises on its own with gentle movements and a balanced diet. You should be patient during this phase as these transient side effects usually go away a few days to a week after the procedure.

SUGGESTED SKINCARE PRODUCTS AND ROUTINES

Establishing a customized skincare regimen is essential for preserving skin health and maximizing outcomes after a non-surgical facelift. It should consist of mild cleansing with a pH-balanced cleanser, followed by the use of hydrating and nourishing serums and moisturizers.

Products with antioxidants and hyaluronic acid can help restore moisture and shield your skin from environmental damage.

To protect your skin from UV rays, which can hasten the aging process and counteract the benefits of your facelift, you should also use a high-SPF sunscreen every day. To prevent irritation during the initial healing phase, stay away from harsh chemicals and abrasive exfoliants.

A skincare specialist or dermatologist can offer customized recommendations based on your skin type and unique post-procedure needs, ensuring optimal outcomes and skin health.

RESCHEDULED VISITS AND PROGRESS TRACKING

Following a non-surgical facelift, it is essential to schedule follow-up appointments to track healing progress, address any concerns, and receive recommendations for further care or adjustments from your healthcare provider.

These appointments also help to identify potential problems early on and make sure you are following your recovery and skincare regimen.

Follow-up visits are an excellent time to discuss any changes or concerns you may have had since your procedure; your healthcare provider may perform additional treatments or adjustments based on your healing progress and desired outcomes. These appointments also provide you with advice on how to maintain results and optimize long-term skin health through continued care and support from your healthcare team.

MODIFICATIONS TO LIFESTYLE FOR EXTENDED RESULTS

One way to extend the benefits of your non-surgical facelift is to make lifestyle changes that will have a substantial impact on skin health and general well-being. You should prioritize regular exercise to improve circulation and promote overall vitality, which will help you look younger and have a radiant complexion. You should also adopt a balanced diet rich in vitamins, minerals, and antioxidants to support cellular repair and regeneration, which will enhance the effects of your procedure.

In addition, getting enough sleep and controlling your stress levels is essential for skin renewal and preserving that youthful glow. Using relaxation methods like yoga or meditation can help lower stress hormones that cause premature aging. Wearing protective clothing and using skincare products with UV protection can help prevent excessive sun exposure and environmental pollutants, which will further protect your skin's integrity and the longevity of your facelift results.

You can reap the full benefits of your non-surgical facelift and experience long-lasting improvements in skin tone, texture, and elasticity by incorporating these lifestyle changes into your daily routine. A holistic approach to well-being along with consistent care guarantees that your investment in skin rejuvenation pays off in the long run and improves your quality of life overall.

CHAPTER SEVEN

POSSIBLE DANGERS AND ISSUES

TYPICAL DANGERS OF NON-SURGICAL FACELIFTS

Even though non-surgical facelift procedures are generally safe, there are some inherent risks that patients should be aware of before undergoing treatment.

These risks include the possibility of infection, although this is rare when procedures are performed in a sterile environment by qualified practitioners using proper techniques. Common risks include temporary swelling, bruising, and redness at the injection site or treatment site. These effects typically subside within a few days to a week but can be distressing for patients immediately after the procedure.

While asymmetry or irregularities in the treated area can occur, particularly if the injectable filler is not evenly distributed or if there is migration of the filler material, these issues are important to consider for anyone considering a non-surgical facelift. Another common risk is allergic reactions to injectable fillers or other substances used in non-surgical facelifts. Patients should disclose any known allergies to their healthcare provider before treatment to mitigate this risk.

INDICES OF DIFFICULTIES AND WHEN TO GET MEDICAL ASSISTANCE

Non-surgical facelifts are very popular and relatively safe, but they can sometimes result in medical complications that need to be addressed. Infection signs, like increased redness, warmth, or pus at the injection site, should be reported to a healthcare provider as soon as possible. Complication signs include severe or persistent pain, excessive swelling, or bruising that does not get better over time.

A rare but serious allergic reaction or vascular compromise could be indicated by sudden changes in vision, dizziness, or difficulty breathing. Patients should also keep an eye out for any lumps, nodules, or skin discoloration that develops in the treated area, as these may also require evaluation by a healthcare professional.

REDUCING HAZARDS WITH APPROPRIATE METHODS AND FOLLOW-UP

Patients can lower their risks by selecting a qualified and experienced provider with a history of safe and effective treatments.

Practitioners should follow proper technique and hygiene standards during treatment, which include using sterile instruments, sanitizing the skin before injections, and making sure the injectable filler is administered in appropriate quantities and depths.

To minimize risks and maximize outcomes, post-procedure instructions—which may include avoiding physically demanding activities, applying ice packs to reduce swelling, and taking prescribed medications as directed—must be carefully followed by patients.

Follow-up appointments with the healthcare provider enable regular monitoring of the procedure's progress and early detection of any potential complications.

RECOGNIZING UNCOMMON BUT POTENTIAL SIDE EFFECTS

Vascular compromise—where the filler unintentionally blocks blood flow to surrounding tissues, potentially resulting in tissue damage or necrosis—is one of the rare but potentially harmful side effects of non-surgical facelift procedures that patients should be aware of.

This complication emphasizes the need for prompt treatment from qualified practitioners who can identify and manage such issues.

Patients should discuss these potential risks with their healthcare provider during the consultation phase so that they can make an informed treatment decision. An additional uncommon but serious adverse outcome is the migration of filler material to unintended areas, which can result in asymmetry or distortion of facial features. There have also been isolated reports of delayed inflammatory reactions or granulomas forming in response to certain types of fillers.

THE RIGHTS OF PATIENTS AND LEGAL CONSIDERATIONS

Legally speaking, patients undergoing non-surgical facelift procedures are entitled to certain protections and rights. These include the right to informed consent, which requires the healthcare provider to fully disclose all potential risks, benefits, and treatment alternatives before receiving the patient's consent; the right to privacy and confidentiality of their medical information; and the right to refuse treatment or seek a second opinion.

Before having any cosmetic procedure, patients should confirm the qualifications and licensure of their healthcare provider. They should also ask to see before-and-after photos of past patients and learn about the provider's experience with non-surgical facelift techniques. If a complication arises or the procedure doesn't go as planned, patients have the right to pursue legal action if they believe negligence or malpractice occurred, though these cases are uncommon when procedures are carried out by licensed professionals in accredited facilities.

CHAPTER EIGHT

FINANCIAL CONSIDERATIONS AND COST ANALYSIS

CALCULATING EXPENSES USING THE SELECTED PROCESS AND SUPPLIER

Understanding the costs of a non-surgical facelift starts with learning about the range of procedures that are available and how much they cost. Costs can differ significantly based on the type of treatment, the provider's experience, and the location. For example, dermal fillers and laser treatments may have different pricing structures depending on the quantity of product used or the number of sessions required. It is important to speak with several providers to obtain a thorough understanding of pricing in your area.

A thorough cost breakdown should be requested during your initial consultation to prevent any unpleasant surprises later on. Some providers may offer package deals for multiple sessions or combine treatments, which can affect overall costs. It's important to factor in not only the procedure itself but also any additional fees such as consultation charges, facility fees, and post-procedure care.

Additionally, reading through patient testimonials and reviews can give you an idea of the caliber of care that various providers offer. Cost is a major consideration, but you should also give top priority to a provider with a solid reputation and a successful track record. With careful investigation and clear pricing information, you can make an educated choice about your non-surgical facelift procedure.

AVAILABLE FINANCING OPTIONS AND INSURANCE COVERAGE

It is important to check with your insurance provider to find out what expenses, if any, are eligible for reimbursement. Non-surgical facelift procedures are generally considered elective and may not be covered by insurance. However, some insurance plans may offer coverage for certain aspects of treatment, such as consultations or tests related to medical necessity.

Before committing to a financing option, it's advisable to make sure it fits within your budget. Many providers offer payment plans or financing through third-party lenders, allowing patients to spread out payments over time. For those without insurance coverage, financing options can help manage the upfront costs of a non-surgical facelift.

Additionally, some providers may provide promotions or discounts for new patients or for booking multiple treatments at once; taking advantage of these opportunities can help lower overall costs. Early in the planning process, inquire about financing and insurance coverage options so that you can make arrangements that work for your specific situation.

SPENDING PLANS FOR TESTS AND PRE-PROCEDURE CONSULTATIONS

To ensure a smooth and successful treatment experience, budget for pre-procedure consultations and tests before having a non-surgical facelift.

Consultations with a provider are usually required to discuss treatment goals and determine your candidacy for specific procedures; the consultation fee may vary depending on the practice and the provider's level of expertise.

Budgeting for these tests guarantees that there are no delays in your treatment timeline and that you are fully prepared for the procedure day. In addition to consultations, some tests or assessments may be necessary before moving forward with treatment. These tests could include skin assessments, allergy tests (if applicable), or blood work to ensure your health and suitability for the chosen procedure.

Budgeting appropriately for pre-procedure consultations and tests will help you approach your non-surgical facelift with clarity and confidence. Some practices may offer package deals that include consultations, tests, and the procedure itself, which can be a cost-effective option. It is advisable to ask about the costs of consultations and tests during your initial inquiry with a provider.

COMPARING THE PRICE OF SURGICAL AND NON-SURGICAL FACELIFT OPTIONS

Several factors need to be considered when comparing the costs of non-surgical facelifts and surgical options. Firstly, non-surgical procedures, like injectables or laser treatments, usually have lower upfront costs than surgical facelifts, which usually involve operating room fees, anesthesia costs, and surgeon fees. Secondly, non-surgical treatments may need to be maintained over time, which can add up over time.

It's important to compare these options based on your desired outcomes, budget, and ability to tolerate downtime. Speaking with both non-surgical and surgical providers can help you better understand the overall costs and benefits of each treatment approach. Surgical facelifts, on the other hand, offer more dramatic and long-lasting results but may require longer recovery times.

Furthermore, it is important to assess how long-lasting the results are when comparing prices. Non-surgical procedures could provide more immediate and little downtime, but surgical facelifts can offer more extensive rejuvenation that lasts for many years. Knowing these distinctions will help you make an educated choice based on your desired appearance and your budget.

UNDERSTANDING CONTRACTS AND BARGAINING FOR PAYMENT PLANS

Managing the financial aspects of a non-surgical facelift requires navigating payment plans and understanding contracts. To accommodate a variety of budgets, many providers offer flexible payment options, such as installment plans or financing through third-party lenders. It's important to carefully review the terms of any payment plan, including interest rates, fees, and repayment schedules, to make sure they are manageable for you.

Contracts should specify the obligations of both the provider and the patient, including expectations for pre-procedure preparations, post-procedure care, and potential outcomes. If there are any clauses or terms that are unclear, don't hesitate to ask the provider for clarification before signing. It's also important to understand the terms of the contract to determine what services are included in the quoted price and any potential additional costs.

You can feel confident in your financial arrangements and concentrate on achieving your desired aesthetic results by openly discussing payment options and contract terms with your provider. By negotiating payment plans and understanding contracts, you ensure transparency and help prevent misunderstandings or surprises during the treatment process.

CHAPTER NINE

ANSWERS TO COMMON QUESTIONS (FAQS)

WHAT AGE IS REQUIRED TO UNDERGO A NON-SURGICAL FACELIFT?

To ensure safety and efficacy, several factors must be taken into account when determining the minimum age for a non-surgical facelift. Most people who are thinking about a non-surgical facelift are in their late 30s or older, which is when fine lines, wrinkles, and mild sagging start to show. Nevertheless, the suitability of a non-surgical facelift depends more on the individual concerns and skin condition than on a rigid age limit. Some younger people in their 20s or 30s may choose preventative treatments or address specific early signs of aging, while older people may want rejuvenation without invasive surgery.

Before pursuing any non-surgical facelift procedure, it is imperative to have a consultation with a qualified practitioner to evaluate skin elasticity, facial anatomy, and general health. The practitioner will assess skin quality, bone structure, and individual goals to determine whether non-surgical options such as dermal fillers, PDO threads, or laser treatments are appropriate. They will also go over realistic expectations and potential outcomes based on age-related skin changes and desired improvements.

A qualified provider will conduct a thorough assessment, educate on available options, and customize a treatment plan to address specific concerns while ensuring natural-looking results.

By being aware of these factors and speaking with a skilled professional, people can make well-informed decisions about non-surgical facelifts that are tailored to their age and aesthetic goals. When thinking about a non-surgical facelift at any age, it is important to prioritize a practitioner's experience and credentials for safe and effective treatment.

HOW MUCH TIME DO OUTCOMES USUALLY LAST?

Results from a non-surgical facelift can take a variety of lengths of time to show; they can last anywhere from several months to more than a year. Certain treatments have longer-lasting effects than others; dermal fillers, for example, can give immediate volume enhancement that lasts anywhere from six months to two years, depending on the type of filler used and the area treated.

Another well-liked non-surgical option is PDO thread lifts, which stimulate collagen production and can show results over several months that can last up to 1-2 years. Laser treatments, on the other hand, improve skin tone and texture, but they can take multiple sessions to see the best results, and the duration of the effects can vary from 6 months to 2 years, depending on the severity of the treatment and the individual's skin response.

Maintaining the results of a non-surgical facelift requires adhering to the post-procedure care instructions given by your practitioner. These instructions include avoiding excessive sun exposure, using skincare products recommended by your practitioner, and scheduling periodic touch-up treatments as advised. Lifestyle factors such as smoking, stress, and diet can also affect how long the results last. Patients can extend the benefits of their non-surgical facelift treatments by knowing how long they will last and making the necessary maintenance commitments.

ARE FACELIFTS WITHOUT SURGERY PAINFUL?

While pain levels can vary based on an individual's tolerance and the particular treatment selected, non-surgical facelift procedures are intended to minimize discomfort and downtime in comparison to traditional surgical facelifts. The majority of non-surgical facelift techniques use topical numbing creams or local anesthesia to ensure patient comfort during the procedure; for instance, injectable treatments like dermal fillers or PDO threads typically cause minimal discomfort due to the small needles and numbing agents used.

The sensation during these procedures is often described as mild to moderate, with many patients finding the discomfort to be manageable and brief. Patients undergoing laser treatments for skin rejuvenation may experience a mild sensation of heat or tingling, which is generally well-tolerated and can be managed with cooling techniques or adjustments in treatment settings.

Overall, non-surgical facelift procedures are designed to prioritize patient comfort while achieving natural-looking results with minimal pain and downtime. Practitioners may recommend over-the-counter pain relievers and cold compresses to alleviate any post-procedure discomfort. Mild swelling, redness, or bruising at the treatment site may occur after the procedure but typically resolves within a few days to a week.

CAN I HAVE OTHER COSMETIC TREATMENTS DONE IN ADDITION TO NON-SURGICAL METHODS?

To achieve comprehensive facial rejuvenation that is customized to each patient's needs and goals, it is common practice to combine non-surgical facelift methods with other cosmetic procedures. The choice to combine treatments is based on several factors, including the areas of concern, the desired outcomes, and general health considerations. Many patients opt to augment the results of non-surgical facelifts with complementary procedures such as Botox injections for dynamic wrinkle reduction or laser resurfacing for improved skin texture.

Combining treatments can address both volume loss and skin laxity in specific facial areas, such as PDO thread lifts and dermal fillers, which can provide a more comprehensive rejuvenation than either procedure alone. However, before combining treatments, it is imperative to speak with a qualified practitioner who can evaluate candidacy, go over potential synergies between procedures, and create a customized treatment plan.

Synergistic non-surgical methods can produce natural-looking results and improve overall facial appearance. The practitioner will assess the patient's skin condition, medical history, and aesthetic goals during the consultation to recommend the most effective combination of procedures.

They will also educate the patient on the expected outcomes, recovery process, and potential side effects associated with the combined treatments.

HOW CAN I PICK A QUALIFIED PROFESSIONAL?

To ensure safe, effective, and satisfying results from non-surgical facelift procedures, it is important to choose a qualified practitioner. A few things to look for in a provider are credentials, aesthetic medicine experience, and community reputation. First, look up practitioners who specialize in non-surgical facelift techniques like dermal fillers, PDO threads, or laser treatments.

Check the practitioner's credentials and training history to make sure they are certified and licensed to perform cosmetic procedures. Seek affiliations with respectable professional associations such as the American Society of Plastic Surgeons or the American Academy of Dermatology, which maintain high standards of practice and patient care. Examine before-and-after photos and patient testimonials to determine the practitioner's level of skill and the caliber of the results.

A qualified practitioner will perform a thorough assessment of your skin condition, customize a treatment plan based on your needs, and provide realistic expectations for results. Schedule a consultation with potential providers to discuss your goals, ask about their approach to treatment, and assess their communication style and willingness to address your concerns.

CHAPTER TEN

SELECTING A CLINIC AND PROVIDER

EXAMINING THE QUALIFICATIONS AND EXPERIENCE OF PROFESSIONALS

To ensure safety and efficacy when contemplating non-surgical facelift methods, you must investigate the credentials and experience of practitioners. Start by confirming the practitioners' qualifications, such as their medical degrees and specialized training in aesthetic procedures; look for certifications from reputable boards and memberships in professional organizations related to cosmetic surgery or dermatology; experience greatly influences expertise; ask about the practitioner's years of experience performing non-surgical facelifts and their success rate with patients who are similar to you.

This research phase helps to identify practitioners who not only have the required qualifications but also uphold a positive reputation within the community.

In addition, explore the practitioner's reputation by looking for reviews and testimonials from prior patients. Online platforms, such as review websites and social media pages, can provide valuable insights into patient experiences. Pay attention to feedback regarding the practitioner's bedside manner, communication skills, and overall satisfaction with results.

ASSESSING PATIENT REVIEWS AND CLINIC FACILITIES

The next step is to assess the clinic where the non-surgical facelift will be done. If at all possible, stop by the clinic in person to see how organized, clean, and equipped it is with modern equipment. A well-maintained clinic with cutting-edge technology can make treatment safer and more comfortable. You should also pay attention to the atmosphere and the professionalism of the staff, as these aspects can affect how satisfied you are with the procedure as a whole.

Beyond evaluating the physical space, take into account patient reviews and testimonials that are unique to the clinic. Testimonials from previous clients can offer valuable information about wait times, flexibility with scheduling, and the general vibe of the clinic. Positive reviews that emphasize the staff's attentiveness and efficiency can reassure you when selecting a specific clinic for your non-surgical facelift; on the other hand, unsettling reviews should make you look into the clinic further or think about going to another one.

MAKING THE CORRECT INQUIRIES IN THE FIRST CONSULTATIONS

To obtain relevant information and make an educated decision, you must ask the right questions during your initial consultations with potential practitioners. Begin by finding out which non-surgical facelift techniques are available and how they can address your specific concerns. Talk about the anticipated outcomes of the procedure, including any potential risks or side effects. Identify the practitioner's philosophy regarding patient care, including follow-up appointments and post-procedure support.

Inquire about pricing and any potential additional costs involved, ensuring transparency regarding the financial aspects of the treatment; utilize this opportunity to gauge the practitioner's responsiveness and willingness to address your questions and concerns comprehensively; by asking thoughtful and thorough questions during the consultation, you can better assess whether the practitioner and clinic align with your expectations and needs. It's also important to ask about the practitioner's availability and accessibility in case of emergencies or unexpected concerns following the procedure.

THE SIGNIFICANCE OF PROFESSIONAL ASSOCIATIONS AND CERTIFICATIONS

Professional affiliations and certifications are important indicators of the legitimacy and experience of practitioners offering non-surgical facelift methods. Look for certifications from dermatology or aesthetic medicine-focused boards or organizations; these credentials show that the practitioner has completed extensive training and satisfies specific competency requirements for non-surgical procedures.

Selecting a practitioner with pertinent certifications and active participation in professional affiliations can reassure you about their qualifications and dedication to providing safe and effective treatments. Professional affiliations with reputable organizations demonstrate a commitment to ongoing education and adherence to ethical standards within the field. Check the validity of certifications and memberships by checking with the issuing organizations or visiting their official websites.

MAKING AN INFORMED DECISION AND TRUSTING YOUR INSTINCTS

Choosing the right practitioner for a non-surgical facelift ultimately comes down to following your instincts and making an informed decision. After doing extensive research, visiting clinics, reading reviews, and asking detailed questions during consultations, go with your first instinct regarding the practitioner and clinic that most resonate with you. Take into account aspects like comfort level with the practitioner, confidence in their abilities, and alignment with your expectations and treatment goals.

Before committing to a non-surgical facelift procedure, take your time and carefully consider all the information you have gathered, including credentials, clinic facilities, patient reviews, and the practitioner's approach to patient care. Clarify any remaining doubts or uncertainties. By following your gut and making an informed decision, you can improve your overall experience and raise the possibility that the treatment will yield satisfying results.

CHAPTER ELEVEN

PROSPECTS FOR NON-SURGICAL FACELIFT TRENDS

TECHNOLOGICAL AND TECHNICAL ADVANCEMENTS

Recent technological and procedural developments have revolutionized non-surgical facelift methods, providing safer and more effective alternatives to traditional surgical procedures. One such development is the application of ultrasound and radiofrequency devices, which target specific layers of the skin to achieve lifting and firming effects, stimulating collagen production without requiring incisions.

Additionally, laser technology has advanced to address a variety of skin concerns, such as uneven skin tone, fine lines, and wrinkles. Laser treatments function by stimulating skin regeneration and encouraging the production of new, healthier skin cells.

With the advent of sophisticated injectables like dermal fillers and neurotoxins, non-surgical facelift techniques have also improved. Dermal fillers, like hyaluronic acid-based injectables, restore volume to areas of the face that are sagging or hollowing, giving it a more youthful contour, while neurotoxins, like botulinum toxin (e.g., Botox), temporarily relax facial muscles to smooth out wrinkles and prevent new ones from forming. These injectables are administered by qualified professionals who are knowledgeable about facial anatomy, guaranteeing natural-looking results with little recovery time.

In addition, developments in non-surgical facelifts encompass the improvement of minimally invasive techniques such as thread lifts, which entail the insertion of dissolvable threads beneath the skin to elevate and reinforce drooping tissues. The dissolving nature of the threads induces the production of collagen, which amplifies the lifting effect. These techniques are appropriate for people seeking to revitalize their appearance without resorting to extensive surgery, providing a tailored method of facial contouring and renewal.

NEW DEVELOPMENTS IN NON-INVASIVE FACELIFTING

New developments in non-invasive facial rejuvenation emphasize maximizing natural beauty with minimal downtime and discomfort. One noteworthy development is the emergence of combination therapies, which combine various non-surgical methods to produce comprehensive outcomes. For instance, clinics can provide a package that consists of laser resurfacing for improved skin texture, followed by injectable treatments for wrinkle reduction and volume restoration. This comprehensive approach guarantees that multiple issues are addressed in one session, optimizing results for patients who desire a more youthful appearance.

The personalization of treatments through advanced diagnostics and imaging technologies is another trend that is rapidly gaining traction. Clinicians are now able to assess facial anatomy and tailor treatment plans based on 3D imaging and computer simulations. This personalized approach guarantees that each patient receives recommendations that are specifically tailored to their unique facial structure and aesthetic goals. Preventive treatments are also becoming more and more popular, with younger people actively maintaining the health of their skin to delay the onset of signs of aging.

Improved formulations and delivery methods have led to the continued evolution of non-invasive techniques like chemical peels and microneedling. Chemical peels use mild acids to exfoliate the skin, revealing a smoother and more radiant complexion; these treatments are perfect for people with mild to moderate skin concerns and can be tailored based on skin type and sensitivity. Microneedling stimulates collagen production through tiny needles that create micro-injuries in the skin, promoting healing and rejuvenation.

PROSPECTIVE ADVANCEMENTS IN SKINCARE AND THERAPY CHOICES

The field of regenerative medicine is experiencing growth as stem cell therapies and growth factors are investigated for their rejuvenating properties. These treatments aim to harness the body's natural healing processes to repair and regenerate aging skin, offering long-lasting results without invasive procedures. Research in this area is expanding, paving the way for more advanced and effective anti-aging solutions. Advances in skincare and treatment options that target aging at its source could pave the way for future non-surgical facelifts.

Additionally, skincare diagnostics and treatment planning are being revolutionized by the integration of artificial intelligence (AI) and machine learning. AI algorithms evaluate enormous volumes of data to forecast individual skin responses and suggest customized skincare regimens. This technology not only improves treatment outcomes but also enables ongoing improvement based on real-time patient feedback. Moreover, nutraceuticals and oral supplements that support skin health from within are becoming more and more popular as a complement to topical treatments for comprehensive anti-aging benefits.

Next-generation skincare technology will offer patients enhanced results with minimal risk or discomfort. Examples of innovative delivery systems for skincare ingredients include nanotechnology and microencapsulation, which improve the penetration of active ingredients into the skin, maximizing their effectiveness and reducing potential side effects. For instance, nanoemulsions deliver vitamins and antioxidants deep into the dermis, where they can neutralize free radicals and promote cellular repair.

COMBINING CONTEMPORARY METHODS WITH HOLISTIC APPROACHES

Combining holistic methods with contemporary non-surgical facelift procedures highlights how vital overall health is to attaining youthful, glowing skin.

Holistic approaches, such as nutrition counseling, stress reduction, and lifestyle modifications, are vital to preserving skin health and improving treatment results. For example, a well-balanced diet high in antioxidants and vital nutrients promotes collagen production and skin regeneration, which amplifies the benefits of non-invasive procedures.

Acupuncture treatments can stimulate facial muscles and improve skin elasticity, contributing to a more lifted and toned appearance over time. Herbal supplements and topical preparations with natural ingredients offer gentle yet effective solutions for skin rejuvenation, harnessing the power of botanical extracts and plant-based antioxidants. Additionally, holistic skincare approaches incorporate traditional healing practices like acupuncture and herbal medicine, which promote circulation and balance energy flow in the body.

Holistic modalities like lymphatic drainage and facial massage are also beneficial to modern non-surgical facelift techniques because they reduce inflammation, stimulate lymphatic circulation, and improve skin care product absorption. Practitioners can guarantee comprehensive care that addresses both aesthetic concerns and overall skin health by incorporating these techniques into treatment protocols. Holistic approaches also promote a synergistic relationship between inner wellness and outer beauty, enabling individuals to achieve sustainable results through natural and non-invasive means.

CONTINUING EDUCATION AND INITIATIVE IN FACIAL REJUVENATION

A clinic that prioritizes continuing education and makes advanced equipment investments will provide patients with optimal treatment outcomes and patient satisfaction. Remaining informed and proactive in facial rejuvenation requires staying up to date on the latest advancements, research findings, and available treatment options. Education and ongoing training for practitioners ensure that they deliver safe and effective care using state-of-the-art techniques and technologies.

A daily skincare routine that includes cleansing, moisturizing, and sun protection is crucial for maintaining skin health and minimizing the effects of aging. Products enhanced with antioxidants, peptides, and retinoids help repair damage, stimulate collagen production, and prevent future signs of aging. Regular consultations with skincare professionals allow for adjustments to treatment plans based on skin changes and evolving aesthetic goals. In addition, proactive skincare practices at home complement professional treatments and prolong their benefits.

Maintaining open lines of communication with medical professionals encourages a cooperative approach to facial rejuvenation in which patients take an active role in goal-setting and decision-making. Clinics that place a high value on patient education and transparency establish credibility and enable people to make educated decisions about their cosmetic journey.

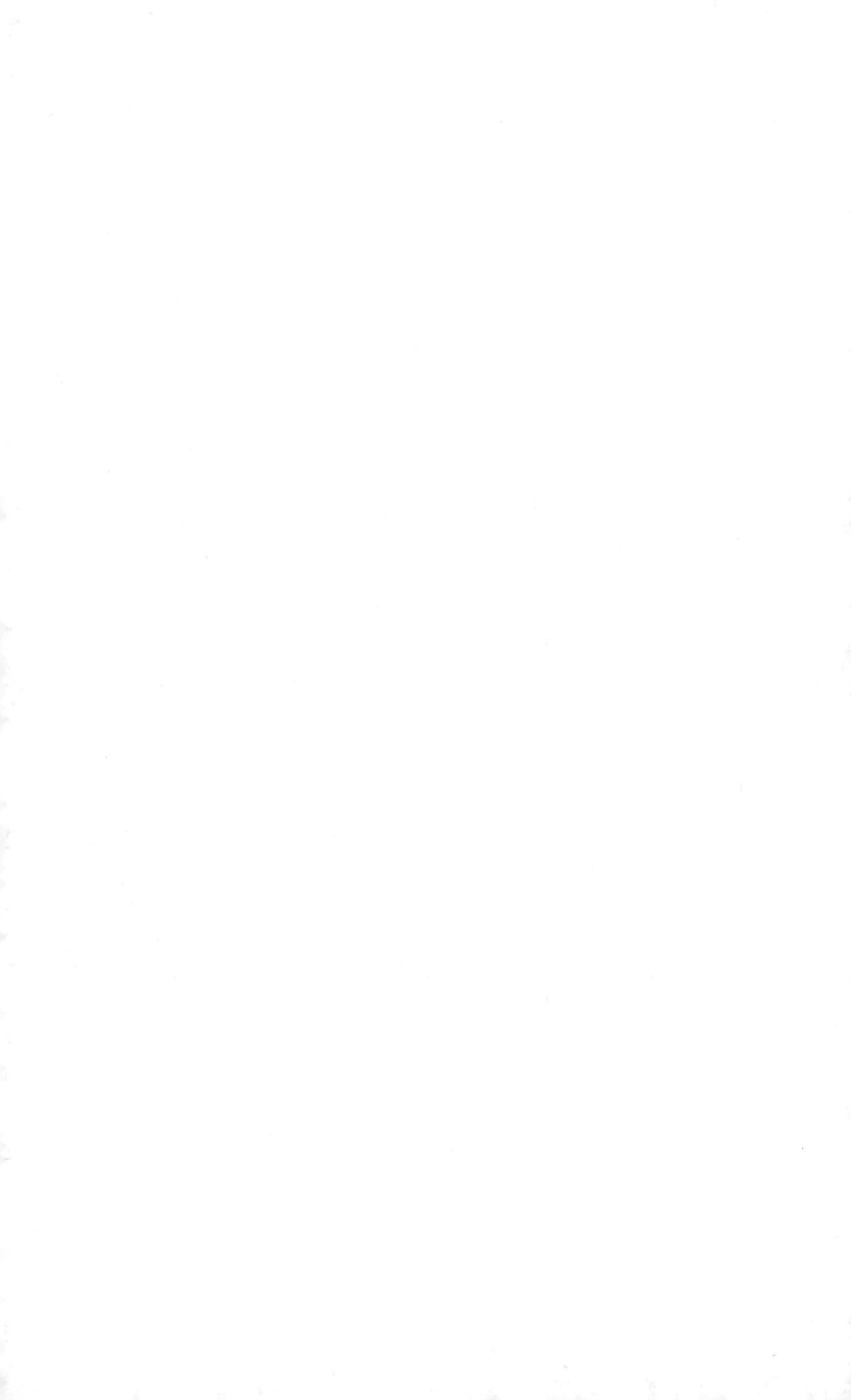

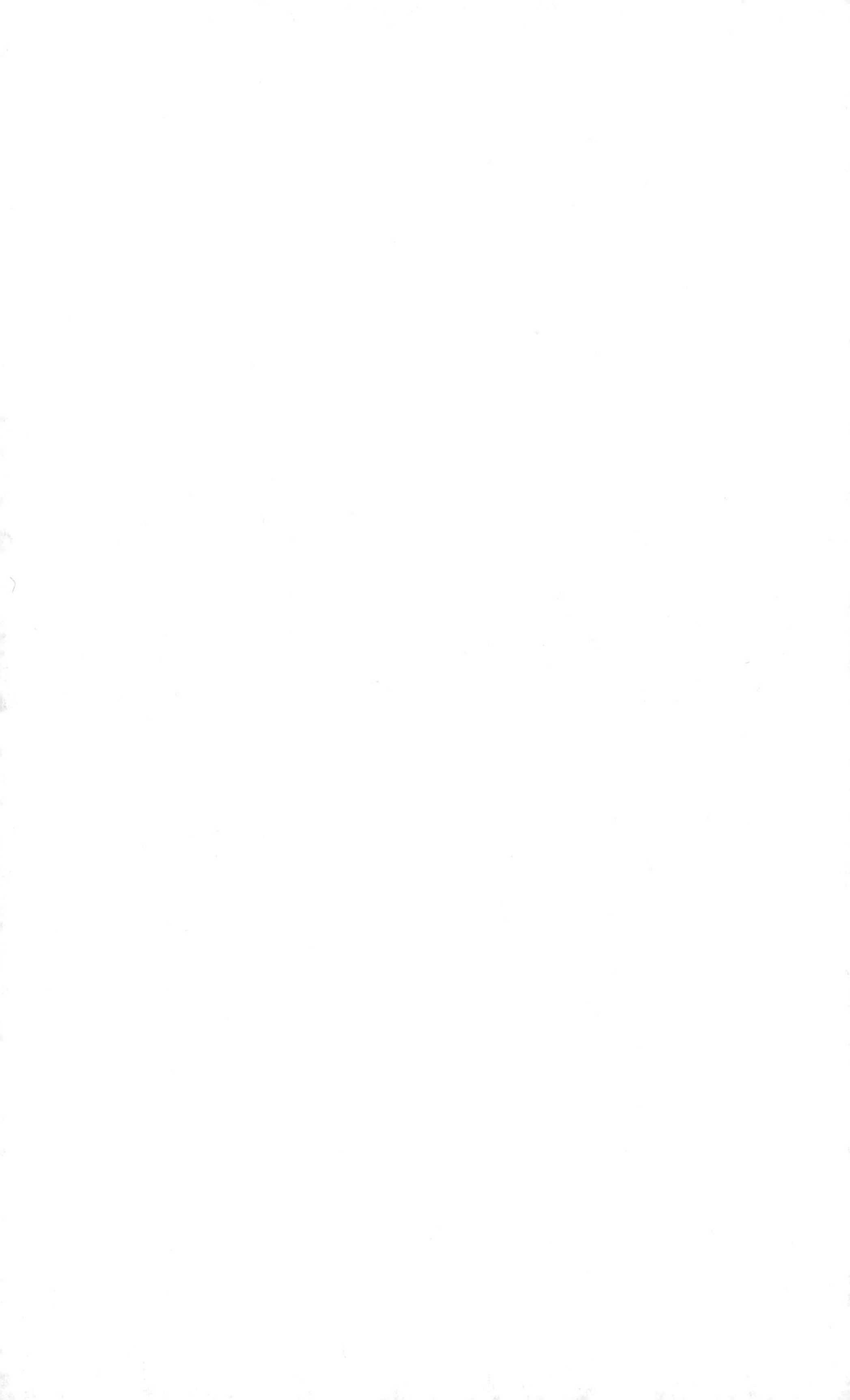